Kyle and his Extra X and Y

Copyright 2014 Regents of the University of Colorado.
All Rights Reserved

Created by Arlene Colvin, Suzanne Hayes, Susan Howell, and Nicole Tartaglia.

All characters appearing in this work are fictitious. Any resemblance to real persons, living or dead, is purely coincidental.

Forward

The inspiration for the creation of this book comes from working with the families of children with X&Y chromosome variations both in the eXtraordinarY Kids Clinic and at family conferences around the world. There were so many times that we handed reading materials and textbook chapters to parents to learn more about their child's condition, while we had nothing to give their smart, curious children standing next to them. Also, parents often ask how to discuss the diagnosis with their child, but feel unprepared and ill-equipped to do so. This book was created to allow boys with XXYY to learn more about their condition, and to facilitate the discussion between parents and their child about the diagnosis of XXYY.

The author, Arlie Colvin, and the illustrator, Suzanne Hayes, have taken a complex topic and created a fantastic story that explains features of XXYY in a way that kids will be able to understand. Kyle's day captures the story of so many boys we see in the clinic--both children and parents will relate to his experiences. Truly understanding the diagnosis of XXYY takes more than a diagram of chromosomes and can't be fully described by a medical textbook, and this book now provides that missing piece. We look forward to using this book as a tool to support boys with XXYY and their families both today and in the years to come.

Nicole Tartaglia, MD

Susan Howell, MS, CGC

eXtraodinarY Kids Clinic
Children's Hospital Colorado
University of Colorado School of Medicine

Recommendations for using this resource.

Many parents of children with X&Y chromosome variations (also called sex chromosome aneuploidy or sex chromosome abnormalties) report feeling unprepared to talk with their child about the diagnosis. Most parents and adult individuals with X&Y chromosome variations say the discussion should happen early in life. It is our hope that this children's book can be used to introduce the topic to young children in an age-appropriate way. This book covers topics pertinent to children such as difficulties in school and visits to the doctor. In writing this story, we did not set out to mention every medical complication that may be experienced by individuals with this condition, but rather to address those which impact young children most.

- This book is intended for children with 48, XXYY between the ages of 5 and 12 but can be read with individuals of any age.
- This is a story that a parent and child should read together.
- Talking about chromosomal variation is not a one-time event. Parents should expect to have many conversations with their child about this topic. This book can help with that discussion.
- Parents should invite their child to ask questions while reading this story. We hope that this story will encourage discussion between parent and child.
- Parents should tailor the book to their own child's maturity level. For instance if parents feel that their child is not ready for a discussion of puberty or infertility, then parts or all of pages 18 and 19 can be skipped.
- We understand that not all boys with 48, XXYY have the same experiences. For instance, not all children will require occupational therapy. It is at the discretion of the parents to decide which details to include or omit for their child.

Enjoy!

"Kyyyyyle!" he hears his mom yell up the stairs. It's time to wake up for school. Sleepy, Kyle shouts to his mother, "I'm coming." Kyle sits up in bed, stretches and yawns. He has a big day ahead of him! As he stands up, he hears another voice in the hallway -- this time it's his sister. "Come on, Kyle! You're going to make me late again!" Kyle leaves his room and heads downstairs. "I'm awake," he grumbles.

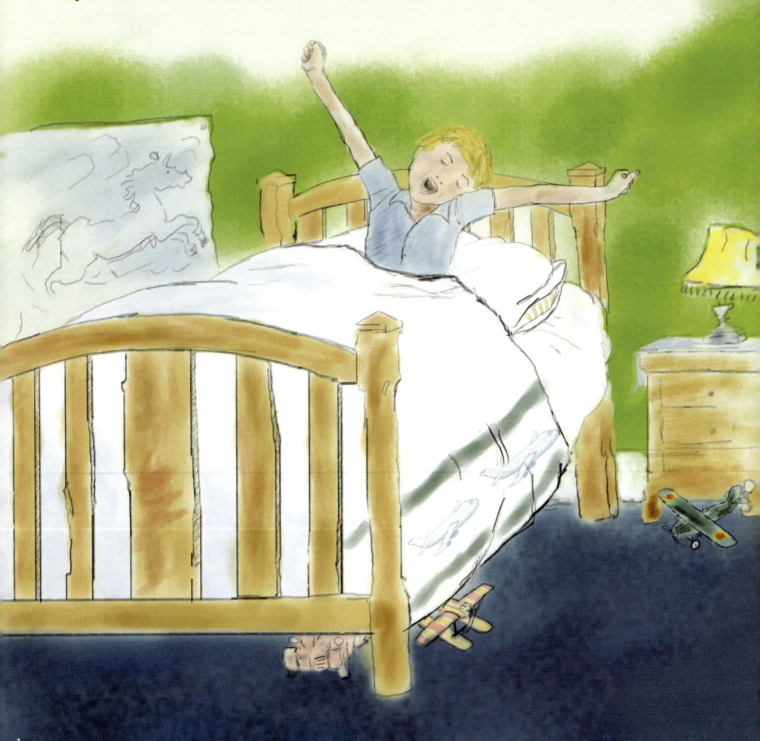

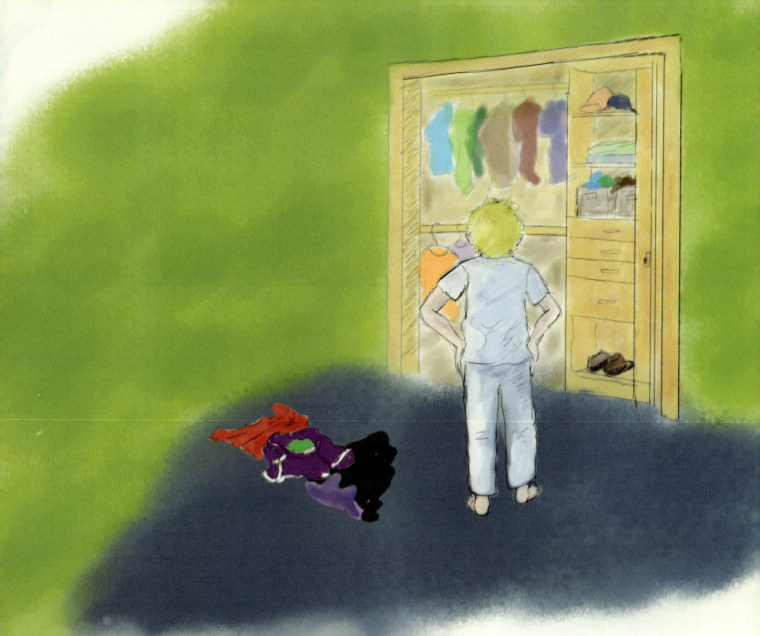

Kyle needs to get ready fast. He gobbles down his cereal and ignores his sister's mean looks from across the table. As he runs back upstairs, his mom yells, "Don't forget to brush your teeth!" Kyle hates brushing his teeth.

He has to get dressed, but it's hard to decide what to wear. Sometimes his clothes feel weird on his skin. He sees his model airplanes and wishes he could play with them. "Kyle! Come on," he hears his sister yell. "Coming, Meg!" he yells back. He grabs his backpack and runs downstairs.

On the way to school, Kyle sits in the backseat while his mom and sister talk about something silly. Kyle stares out the window. He is still upset about how Megan yelled at him that morning. "She doesn't get it," he thinks. "Megan doesn't understand that I have to do things my own way." You see, Kyle is a little different. Kyle has extra chromosomes. He has a condition called XXYY.

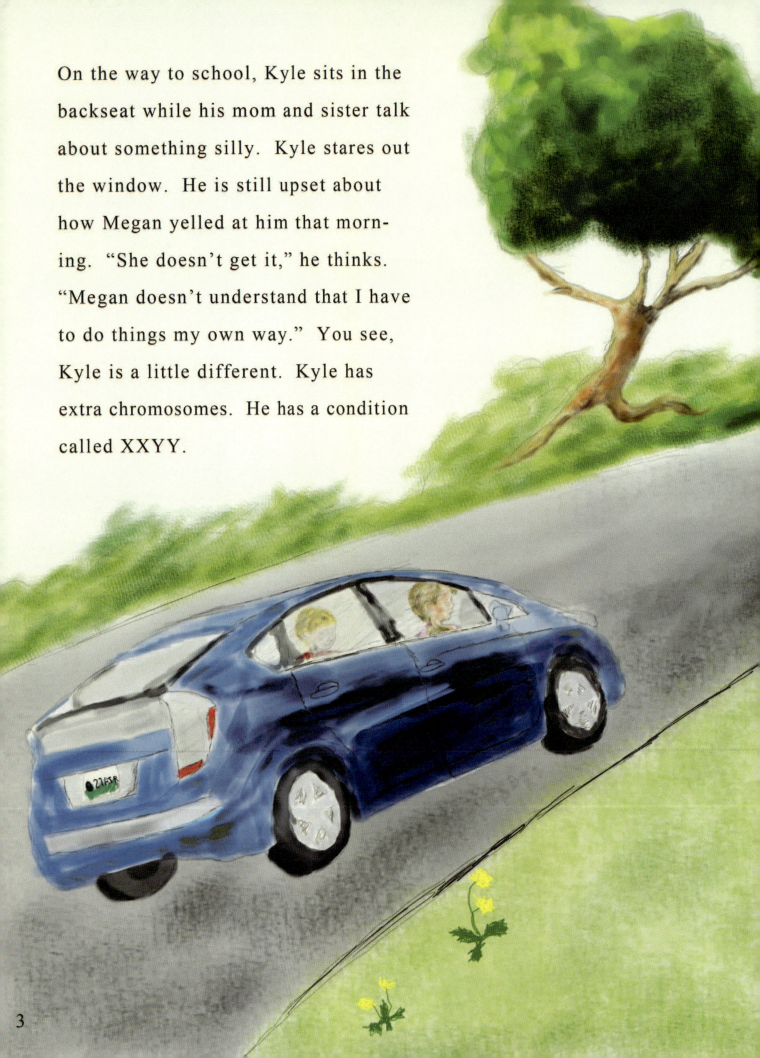

It all starts with genes. These genes are not the jeans you wear. These are the ones that run in families. Genes are in every cell of the body. They are the instructions that tell the body how to grow, what to look like and how to think and act. Genes are important and everyone has them, lots of them! Genes make people unique and different from one another. Without genes, people would be just faceless, brainless blobs of goo!

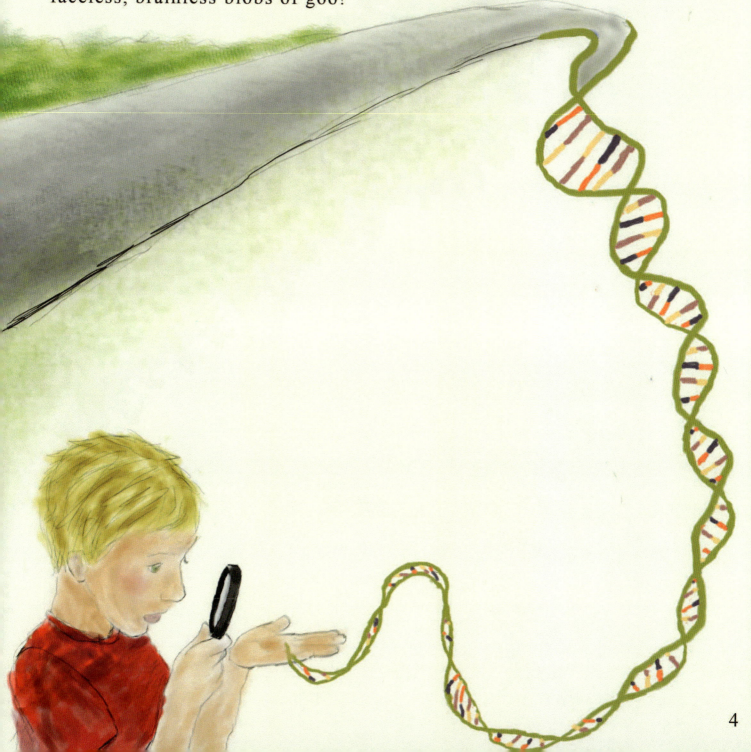

In the body, genes come in bundles called chromosomes. A chromosome holds a bundle of genes, just like a book holds a bundle of pages. There are too many genes to have just one chromosome, so people usually have 46 chromosomes to hold all of their genes. Chromosomes and genes are there from the beginning, when a baby is made. Half of the chromosomes come from your mom and the other half come from your dad. That's why kids look and act a little bit like both of their parents.

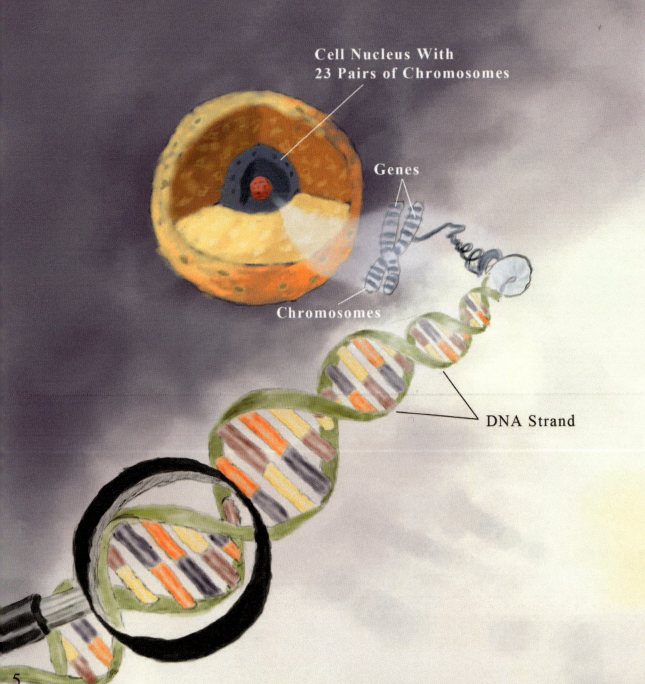

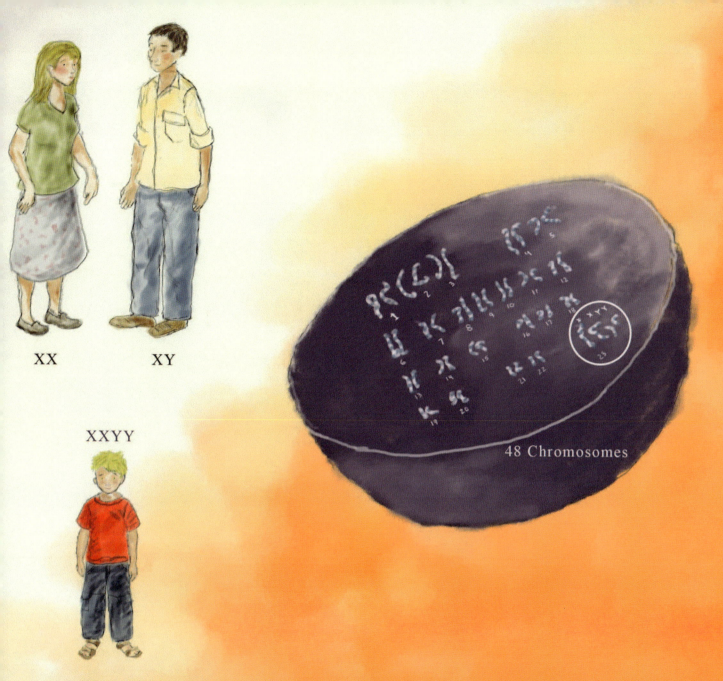

48 Chromosomes

XX   XY

XXYY

Usually, people have 46 chromosomes. Two chromosomes, the X and the Y, are different from the rest. It's these X and Y chromosomes that make boys and girls different. Girls have only X chromosomes, but boys have an X chromosome and a Y chromosome. It's that Y chromosome that makes boys look like boys. Kyle is a boy who is a little different. He was born with an extra X and Y chromosome. So instead of having just one X and one Y like most boys, Kyle has two Xs and two Ys.

When a boy has two Xs and two Ys, like Kyle, it's called XXYY. Having an extra X and Y means Kyle has extra genes in his body.

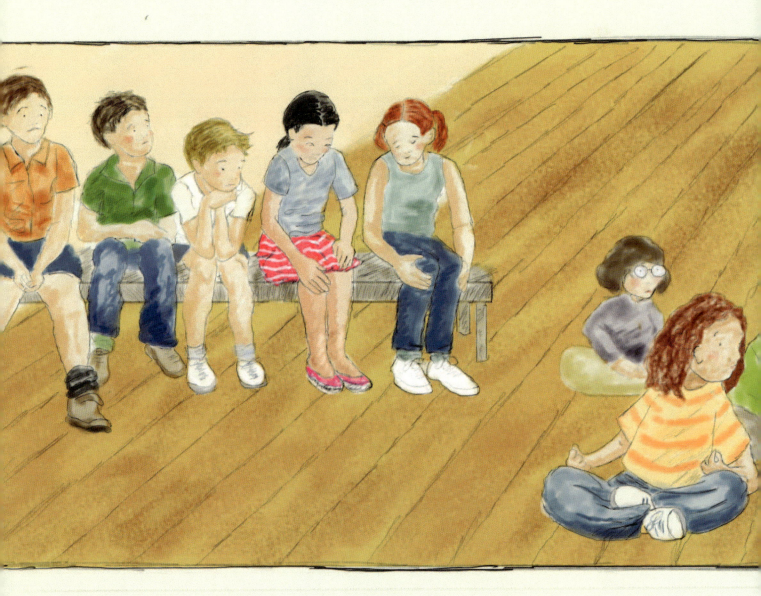

XXYY isn't a sickness like a cold that you can catch from other people. Kyle was just born with an extra X and Y. He isn't the only boy with XXYY either. There are lots of other boys with XXYY. Some of them have the same challenges as Kyle but some don't. Kyle is not ashamed of his extra X and Y. That's just the way he is. He was made with blond hair, green eyes, smelly feet and an extra X and Y!

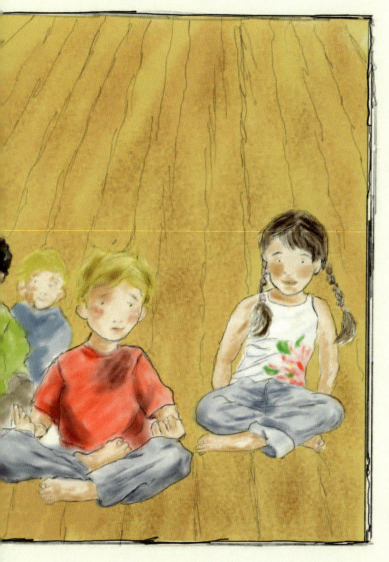

No one can tell he has XXYY just by looking at him. He looks just like the other boys. But inside his brain, sometimes his extra X and Y make him feel different. Sometimes having an extra X and Y can make things harder for him, like reading or school work. That's what Megan doesn't understand. She doesn't get that Kyle is different. He has an extra X and Y and that means he has to do things a different way sometimes.

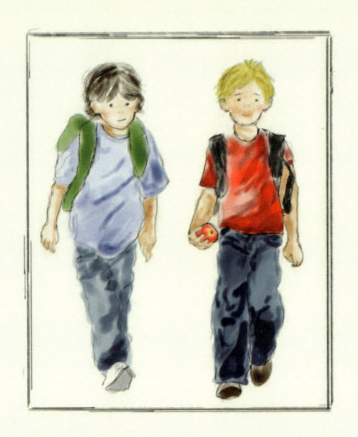

Kyle's mom drives up to his school. He hops out of the car and sees other boys in his class. "Bye, Mom." He catches up with his friend Sam. They walk to class and talk about their weekends. Sam went to the zoo and saw a big giraffe. The boys talk and laugh together. Kyle wants to tell Sam about the time he went to the zoo, but before he can put the words together, he is talking about something else. Oh well. Kyle listens and laughs along with his friend.

The boys go into their classroom and find their seats. Kyle and his friends have special education for some of their subjects to get extra help. It can be hard for Kyle to learn and remember things. He gets bored and wiggles around in his chair.

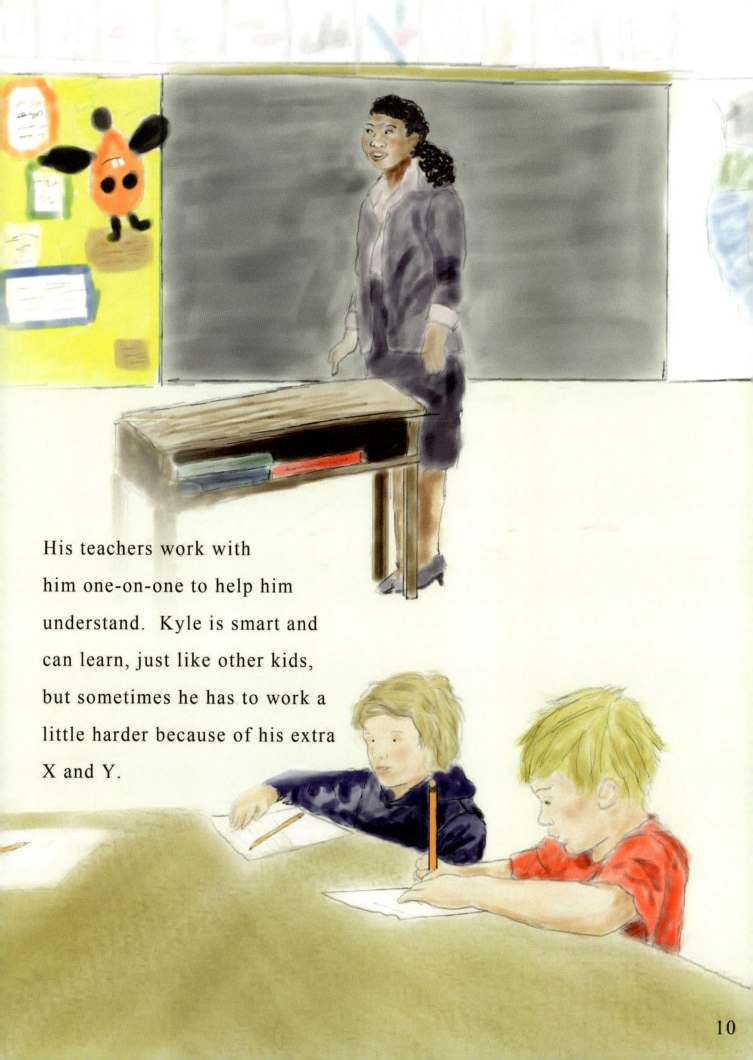

His teachers work with him one-on-one to help him understand. Kyle is smart and can learn, just like other kids, but sometimes he has to work a little harder because of his extra X and Y.

After lunch, Kyle leaves his class to see his speech therapist. His speech therapist helps him learn to talk more easily. Sometimes people talk too fast and he can't keep up, or he blurts out things he's not supposed to say. Other times, it's like a word gets caught in his brain, like when he wanted to talk about the zoo. In speech therapy Kyle practices saying these words. The more he practices, the better he gets!

Kyle meets with an occupational therapist at school too. Occupational therapy helps Kyle practice using his hands to do things that are hard for him, like handwriting and buttoning. He likes to work on his drawings. Kyle imagines all sorts of things to draw. He is the best artist in his whole class! And the more he practices, the better he gets!

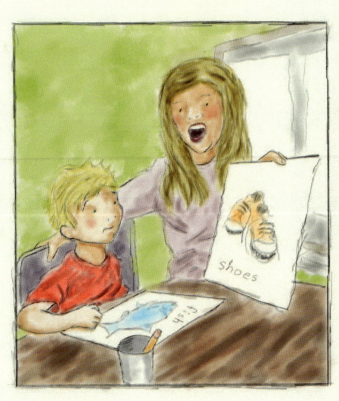
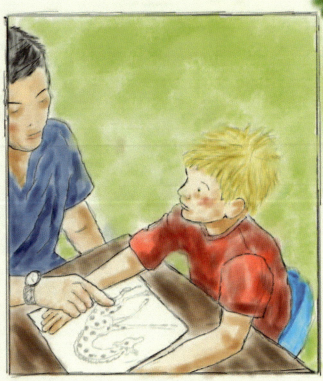

The school bell rings -- recess! He likes taking a break from class and being outside. He and Sam go to the usual spot where they play on the playground. Kyle looks up and sees two boys playing tag, and they are running towards him! Nervous and breathing hard, Kyle is glad when the boys swerve just before running into him. "Hey! Watch it!" Sam yells. It takes a while for Kyle to calm down. He feels overwhelmed by the noise of everyone running around. He walks away from the others to sit by himself and calm down. He closes his eyes and catches his breath. That's better.

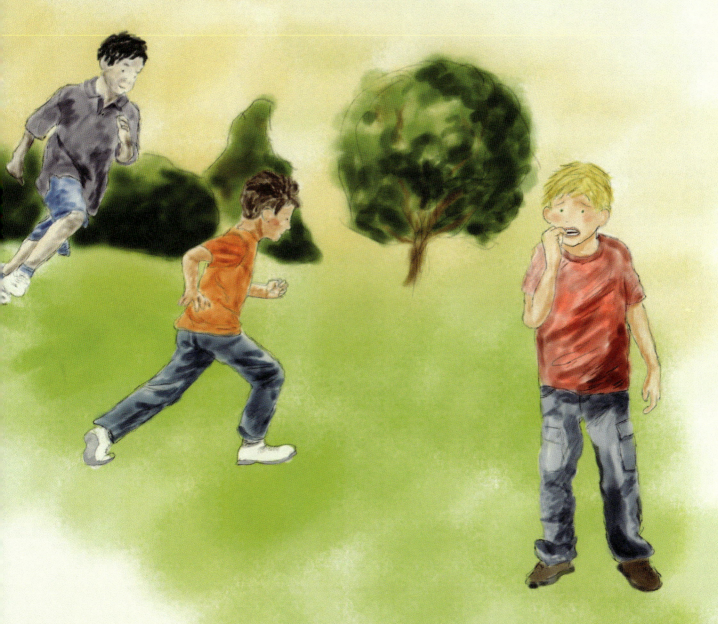

Ring! "Ah, man. Back to class, guys," his friend Sam says. It is harder for Kyle to concentrate after lunch. He takes medication to help him pay attention, but it's tough at the end of the day. Kyle tries to listen to his teacher. It is easier to pay attention when they learn interesting things or get to use the computer. Today the teacher is talking about something boring. He starts to look around and think about something else. The bell finally rings and Kyle snaps back to reality. "See you tomorrow, class," his teacher says as the students get their stuff to go home.

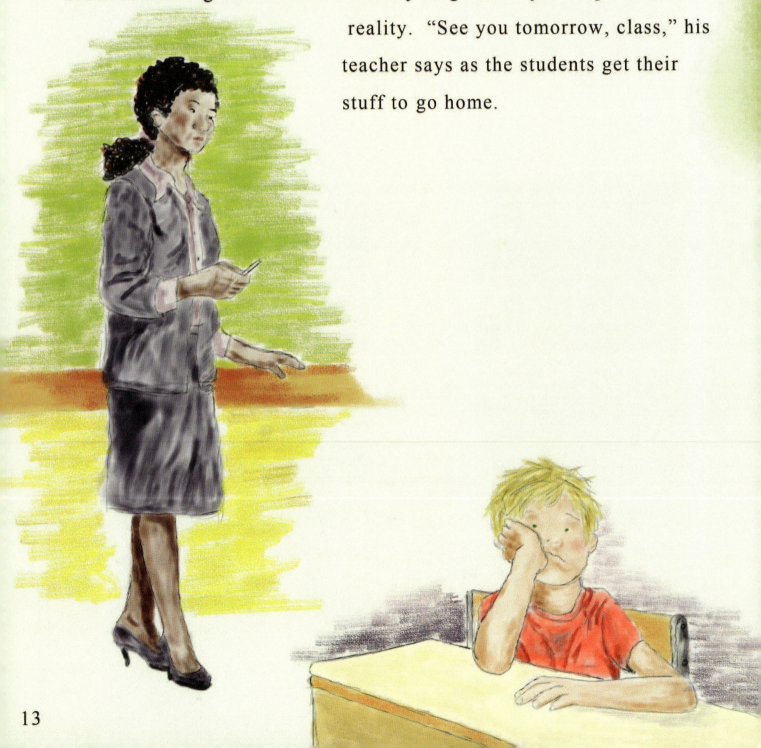

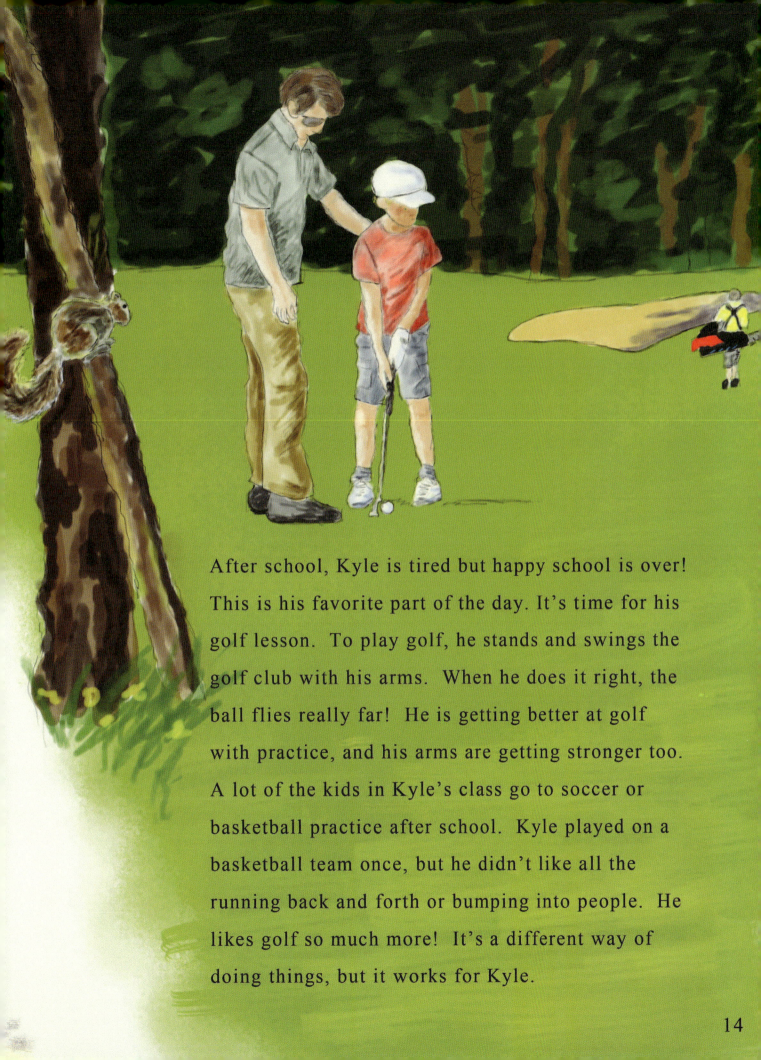

After school, Kyle is tired but happy school is over! This is his favorite part of the day. It's time for his golf lesson. To play golf, he stands and swings the golf club with his arms. When he does it right, the ball flies really far! He is getting better at golf with practice, and his arms are getting stronger too. A lot of the kids in Kyle's class go to soccer or basketball practice after school. Kyle played on a basketball team once, but he didn't like all the running back and forth or bumping into people. He likes golf so much more! It's a different way of doing things, but it works for Kyle.

Tired from golf practice, Kyle walks to the parking lot. His mom is picking him up to take him to his doctor's office. He sees her waving from her car. He smiles and waves back. "Hi, Mom," Kyle says. She starts the car and says, "Hi, honey. How was your day?" Kyle says, "Good." She asks him questions about his day, but he has trouble remembering the details. When he looks inside his backpack he finds the homework he forgot to turn in. "Uh-oh."

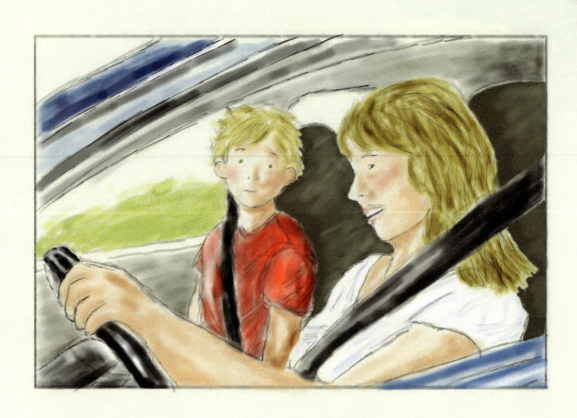

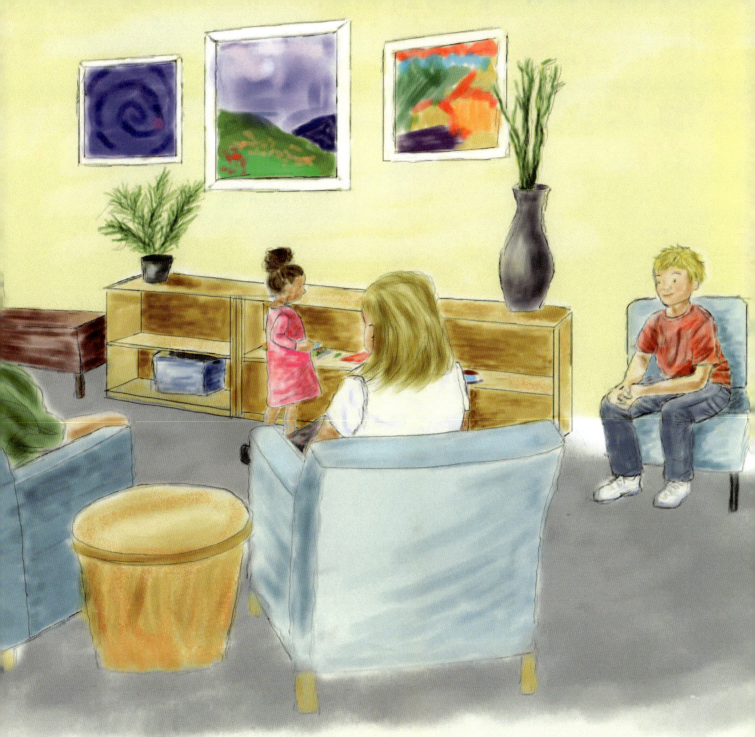

When Kyle and his mom get to the doctor's office, they sit in the waiting room. Kyle stares at the paintings on the wall. "These paintings are ugly," he tells his mom with a laugh. "Kyle, don't be rude," she says, but she laughs too. Kyle has been in this waiting room many times before. Since Kyle has an extra X and Y, he has to go to the doctor a little more than other kids. He doesn't go to the doctor because he is sick; he goes so the doctor can make sure he is healthy.

Finally, the nurse takes them back to the exam room. Kyle sits on the doctor's table. The doctor comes in. She looks at his body, listens to his heart and looks into his ears. She pushes on his stomach which makes him laugh. "That tickles!" The doctor asks, "Kyle, do you know why you have to come to the doctor?" He takes a second to think. "My extra X and Y?" "That's right, Kyle. Boys with XXYY can be tall and need extra help in school. They can sometimes have tremors that make their hands shake or elbows that don't straighten all the way. Boys with XXYY usually need medicine from a doctor to help them during puberty when their bodies change," the doctor explains.

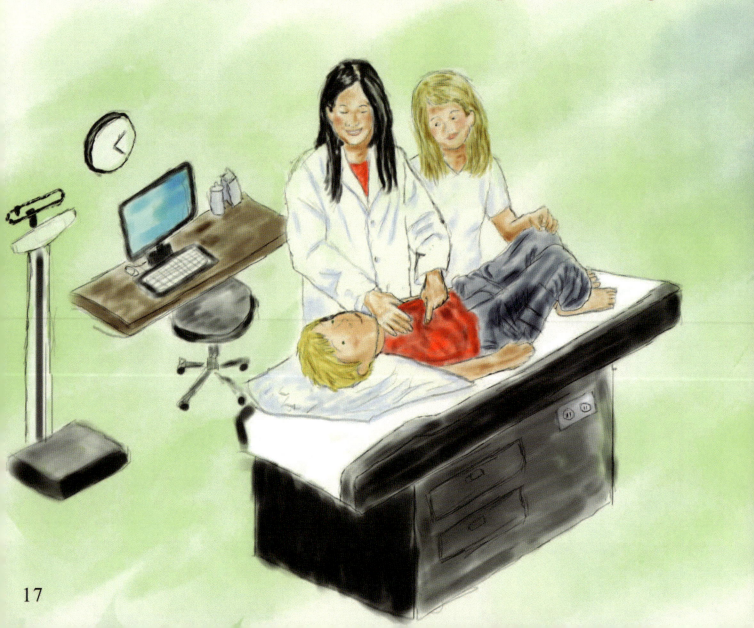

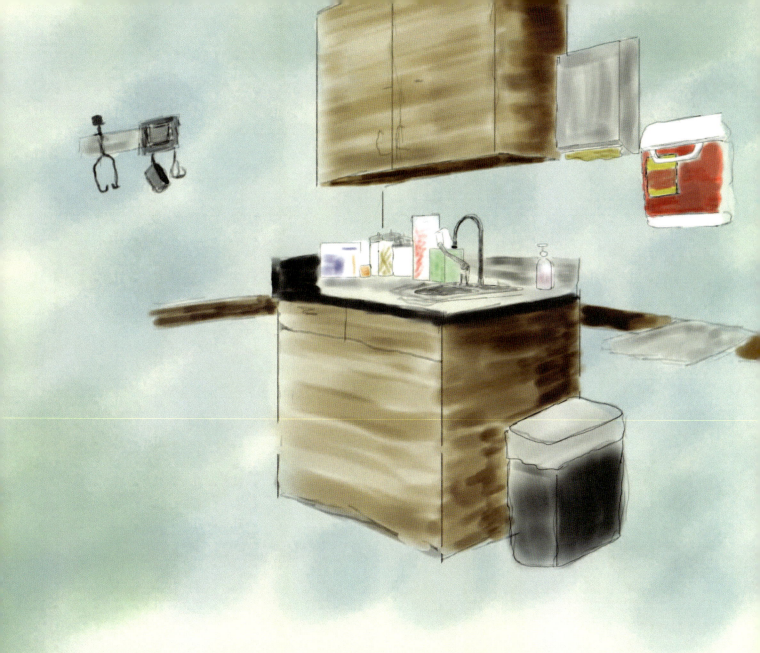

When Kyle is a little older, his doctor will check if he needs a medicine called testosterone to help his body go through puberty. Puberty is when a boy becomes a man. His muscles will get bigger and his voice will get deeper. Most boys go through puberty without the help of a doctor, but since Kyle has XXYY, his body doesn't make enough testosterone to go through puberty. When Kyle is older, the doctor might give him the testosterone medicine to help his body change during puberty like other boys. It's a different way of doing things, but it works for Kyle.

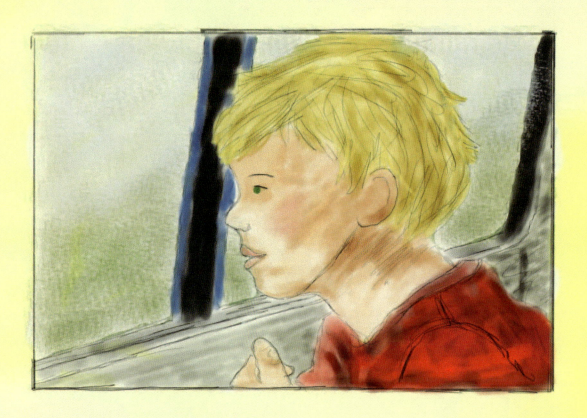

On the way home, Kyle stares out the car window and thinks about the future. Kyle is not sure what he wants to be when he grows up. There are so many things to choose from! He could be a farmer, or a firefighter, or an inventor, or make videogames. He could be an astronaut and live on Mars!

Someday, Kyle might want to be a father and have kids. Kyle can be a father when he grows up, but because of his XXYY, he will need help from a doctor to have children. Or he could adopt a child. It's a different way of doing things, but it works for Kyle.

Back at home, Kyle and his family sit at the table for dinner. Megan blabs about her day. Kyle is too tired to listen. He wants to finish eating so he can play on the computer. Kyle's dad asks him about his day. He takes a second to think. "Um...well..." "Come on, Kyle, I don't have all day," his sister says with a mean grin. Kyle has had enough. Unable to control his feelings, Kyle stands up from the table and yells, "Uhh! I can't stand you. Megan." He runs upstairs to his bedroom and slams his door.

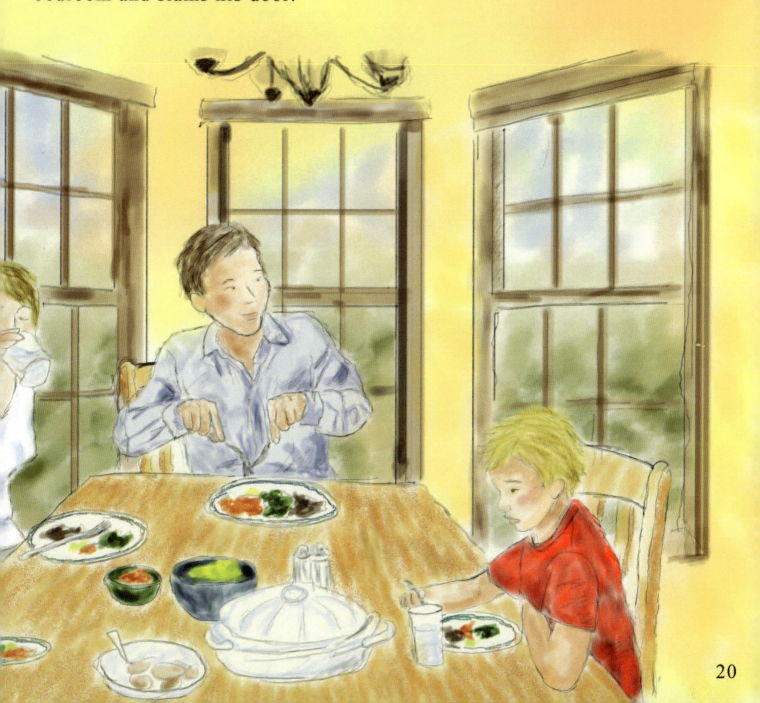

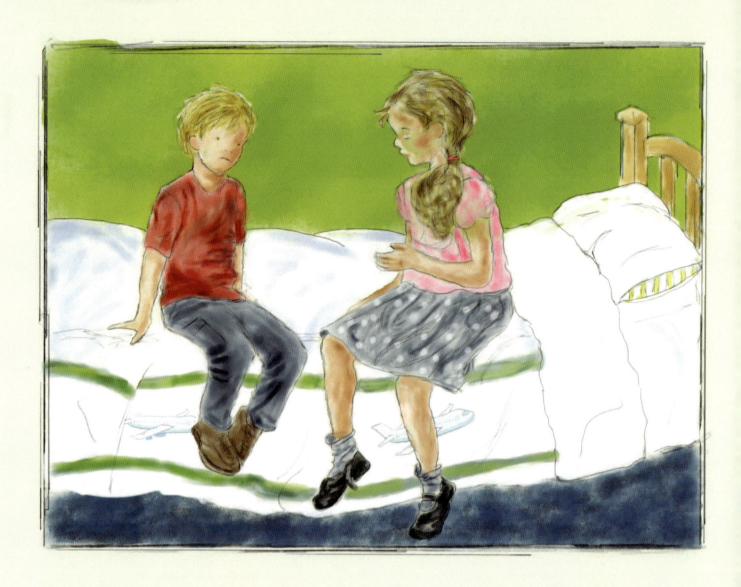

Kyle feels mad and frustrated. "Why does she have to be so mean to me? Doesn't she understand that things aren't as easy for me?" Just then, the door opens. It's Megan. "I came to say sorry," she says. "I didn't mean to make you so mad. I was just teasing." "Megan, you tease me too much. I'm different from you. I have to do things my own way." "I know. I'm sorry. It's important for you to do things your own way," Megan says, "I'll try to be more patient with you. I love you, little brother." Kyle smiles. "Yeah. I love you too, Meg."

It has been a long day. Kyle's mom and dad tuck him into bed. They tell him they love him and close his bedrooom door. As he drifts off to sleep, he thinks about his extra X and Y. Having XXYY is really just a small part of who Kyle is. His extra X and Y make him unique and different, just like all of his talents and traits. His extra X and Y are just two of many, many things that make Kyle who he is. It's a different way of doing things, but it works for Kyle.

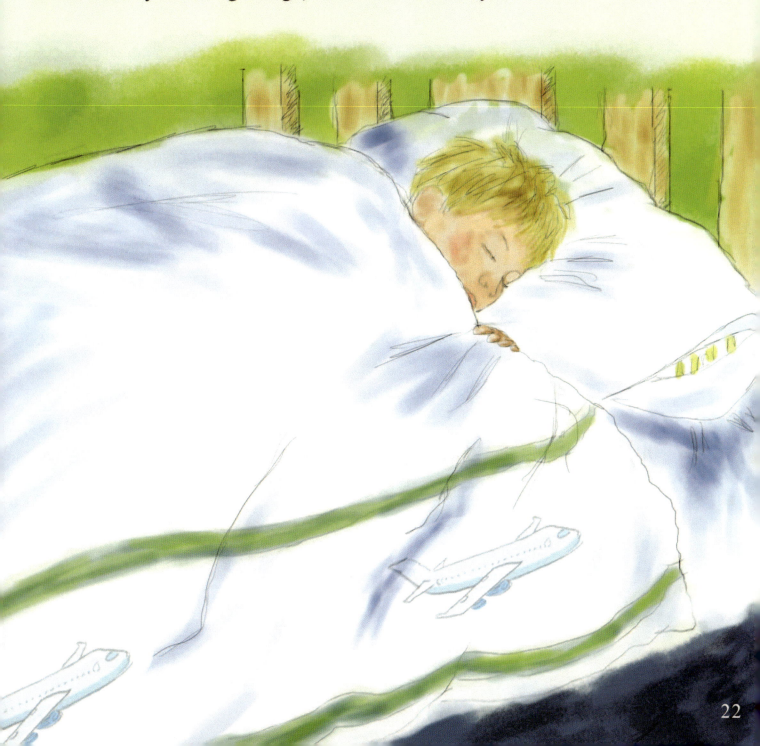

The end.

Acknowledgements

Creating this series of books would not have been possible without the time and dedication of many people who had a hand in bringing it to life.

Firstly, I am indebted to the many parents of children with X and Y chromosome variations who took the time to read the books between the time of their inception through to their final stages. The feedback they provided was so important in helping to craft the stories into ones that so many children will be able to relate to as they flip through these pages. Thank you for your time, wisdom and enthusiam.

I would also like to thank Susan Howell, Dr. Nicole Tartaglia and their colleagues at the eXtraordinarY kids Clinic, whose expertise and advice guided me through the creation of these books. Thank you for your patience, your encouragement and for reading these books almost as many times as I have.

Many thanks go to Suzanne Hayes, the illustrator of this series of books. With her creativity and talents, she was able to take my words and bring them to life in full color images. Her efforts turned my stories into children's books. I appreciate every minute of hard work she devoted to making this project a success.

My editor, Alexa McGuinness, deserves a great deal of thanks for remembering the grammar rules that I didn't and taking the time to read through every line of my books looking for them.

Finally, I would like to thank my family for supporting me in everything that I do and lending names to so many of my characters.

Arlie Colvin
Author

About the author

Born and raised in Muskegon, MI, Arlie Colvin received her Bachelor of Science from the University of Michigan. She attended the University of Colorado Denver to pursue her Master of Science in genetic counseling. She became interested in writing children's books for kids with X and Y chromosome variations while working for the eXtraordinarY Kids Clinic at Children's Hospital Colorado as a graduate student. Arlie enjoys spending time with her family, hiking and painting. She hopes to have a long career as a genetic counselor and children's book author, and impact many people along the way.

Made in the USA
Charleston, SC
18 July 2015